53 PACOIMA

AUG 2 4 2013

W9-AVC-915

EXAM✓PREP

NCLEX®-PN

Wilda Rinehart, Diann Sloan, Clara Hurd

616
R579-2
2011

42045307

NCLEX®-PN Exam Prep

Copyright ® 2011 by Pearson Education, Inc.

All rights reserved. No part of this book shall be reproduced, stored in a retrieval system, or transmitted by any means, electronic, mechanical, photocopying, recording, or otherwise, without written permission from the publisher. No patent liability is assumed with respect to the use of the information contained herein. Although every precaution has been taken in the preparation of this book, the publisher and author assume no responsibility for errors or omissions. Nor is any liability assumed for damages resulting from the use of the information contained herein.

ISBN-13: 978-0-7897-4795-2
ISBN-10: 0-7897-4795-2

Library of Congress Cataloging-in-Publication Data is on file.

Printed in the United States on America

First Printing: May 2011

Trademarks

All terms mentioned in this book that are known to be trademarks or service marks have been appropriately capitalized. Que Publishing cannot attest to the accuracy of this information. Use of a term in this book should not be regarded as affecting the validity of any trademark or service mark.

NCLEX® is a registered trademark of the National Council of State Boards of Nursing, Inc. (NCSBN), which does not sponsor or endorse this product.

Warning and Disclaimer

Every effort has been made to make this book as complete and as accurate as possible, but no warranty or fitness is implied. The information provided is on an "as is" basis. The author and the publisher shall have neither liability nor responsibility to any person or entity with respect to any loss or damages arising from the information contained in this book or from the use of the CD or programs accompanying it.

Bulk Sales

Que Publishing offers excellent discounts on this book when ordered in quantity for bulk purchases or special sales. For more information, please contact

U.S. Corporate and Government Sales

1-800-382-3419

corpsales@pearsontechgroup.com

For sales outside of the U.S., please contact

International Sales

international@pearsoned.com

PUBLISHER
Paul Boger

ASSOCIATE PUBLISHER
David Dusthimer

ACQUISITIONS EDITOR
Betsy Brown

SENIOR DEVELOPMENT EDITOR
Christopher Cleveland

MANAGING EDITOR
Sandra Schroeder

PROJECT EDITOR
Mandie Frank

INDEXER
Tim Wright

PROOFREADER
Leslie Joseph

TECHNICAL EDITORS
Jacqueline Ruckel
MaryEllen Schwarzbek

PUBLISHING COORDINATOR
Vanessa Evans

MULTIMEDIA DEVELOPER
Dan Scherf

DESIGNER
Gary Adair

PAGE LAYOUT
Bronkella Publishing